The Spanish Flu Pandemic of 1918

John Allen

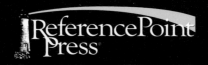

ReferencePoint
Press

San Diego, CA

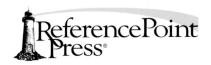

About the Author

John Allen is a writer who lives in Oklahoma City.

© 2022 ReferencePoint Press, Inc.
Printed in the United States

For more information, contact:
ReferencePoint Press, Inc.
PO Box 27779
San Diego, CA 92198
www.ReferencePointPress.com

LIBRARY OF CONGRESS CATALOGING-IN-PUBLICATION DATA

Names: Allen, John, 1957- author.
Title: The Spanish flu pandemic of 1918 / John Allen.
Description: San Diego, CA : ReferencePoint Press, Inc., 2022. | Series: Historic pandemics and plagues | Includes bibliographical references and index.
Identifiers: LCCN 2021005017 (print) | LCCN 2021005018 (ebook) | ISBN 9781678201043 (library binding) | ISBN 9781678201050 (ebook)
Subjects: LCSH: Influenza--History--20th century. | Spanish flu.
Classification: LCC RA644.I6 A45 2022 (print) | LCC RA644.I6 (ebook) | DDC 614.5/1809041--dc23
LC record available at https://lccn.loc.gov/2021005017
LC ebook record available at https://lccn.loc.gov/2021005018

CONTENTS

Important Events During the Spanish Flu Pandemic

March 1918
On March 9, at Fort Riley's Camp Funston in north-central Kansas, Private Albert Gitchell reports to the camp infirmary complaining of severe flu symptoms.

April 1918
An April 5 weekly public health report is the first to mention flu deaths in Haskell County, Kansas.

January 1918
In January, Loring Miner, a local doctor in Haskell County, Kansas, alerts the US Public Health Service about a disturbing outbreak of influenza.

May 1918
On May 22 the largest newspaper in Madrid, Spain, features a front-page article about the country's growing flu outbreak.

September 1918
Beginning on September 7, Camp Devens, a US Army installation near Boston, suffers 100 flu deaths each day.

1917   1918

1917
On April 6 the United States enters World War I on the side of the Allies— Britain, France, and Russia.

May 1918
In May hundreds of thousands of US troops travel across the Atlantic to fight in World War I, carrying the Spanish flu virus to Europe.

September 1918
New York health commissioner Dr. Royal S. Copeland places the entire Port of New York under quarantine on September 12.

August 1918
On August 27 sailors at Boston's Commonwealth Pier show signs of flu infection.

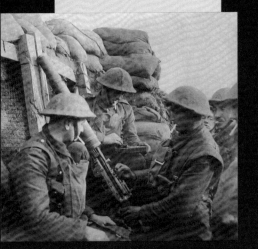

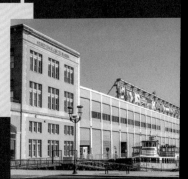

4

September 1918

On September 19 India's major port city of Bombay reports more than 290 flu deaths, the first signs of a devastating outbreak that will kill more than 18 million people in India.

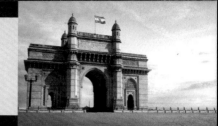

October 1918

With Spanish flu raging across the country, October becomes the deadliest month in US history, with more than 195,000 deaths from influenza and related causes.

November 1918

On November 11 Germany signs an armistice agreement with the Allied powers, ending World War I. Celebrations in the United States, Great Britain, France, and many other countries lead to further spread of Spanish flu.

2005

On October 7 a team of scientists at the Centers for Disease Control and Prevention reconstructs the Spanish flu virus from tissue samples retrieved from flu victims in Alaska.

1919   1920 / 2005

September 1918

Philadelphia officials refuse to cancel a September 28 Liberty Loan parade promoting sales of war bonds. The parade leads to more than 12,000 flu deaths in the city.

September 1918

By September 30, cases of Spanish flu at Camp Devens rise to more than 14,000, with 757 reported deaths, and flu cases have spread to cities across the United States.

June 1919

In June the African nation of Kenya battles an outbreak of Spanish flu that leaves 150,000 dead.

January 1919

In January a third wave of Spanish flu kills thousands more people in the United States and elsewhere in the world.

1920

In mid-January to early February, Japan suffers through Three Weeks of Hell, the culmination of its Spanish flu outbreak. The disease kills more than 450,000 Japanese.

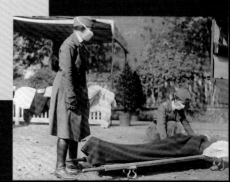

The Deadliest Flu Outbreak in History

Lillian Clayton was exhausted. As chief nurse at Philadelphia General Hospital School of Nursing in October 1918, she found herself on the front lines of the fight against the Spanish flu. Conditions had grown desperate, with all manner of vehicles out front delivering patients by the hour. Most of the infected were dying, and some were already dead. Clayton, age forty-two, had seen influenza outbreaks before, but this illness killed its victims with frightening speed. Moreover, Philadelphia General Hospital was understaffed, with doctors and nurses having gone overseas to care for American troops in World War I. Clayton enlisted her student nurses to fill in where needed. In the packed hospital wards, patients with fever and fluid-filled lungs required constant attention, and more sick people were on the way. Clayton herself was in the midst of her usual forty-eight-hour shift. She took pity on her first-year students, urging them to go home and avoid exposure. However, all volunteered to stay and help. Six of the young nurses contracted the virus and died. Similar scenes played out in cities and towns across the nation. Although overwhelmed, health care professionals like Clayton did their best to stem the tide of illness and death. As nursing historian Elizabeth Hanink notes, "Ultimately, it was the trained nurses, even the beginners, who stuck with the job until the end."[1]

A Months-Long Ordeal

The ordeal for health care workers and stricken communities continued for months. In the United States alone, more than 22 million people were infected with the Spanish flu, and an estimated 675,000 died. An equivalent death toll for today's population in the United States would be 2.1 million people. Experts believe the virus killed 50 million to 100 million people worldwide. "The 1918 influenza pandemic was the deadliest event in all of human history," says David M. Morens, a scientist at the National Institute of Allergy and Infectious Diseases. "It killed more people than any war, any pandemic, the Black Death, AIDS, you can pick your terrible event."[2]

> "Ultimately, it was the trained nurses, even the beginners, who stuck with the job [of treating Spanish flu patients] until the end."[1]
>
> —Elizabeth Hanink, nursing historian

Despite the horrific death toll, some historians consider the Spanish flu to be the forgotten pandemic. Occurring at the end of World War I, the disease was overshadowed by the bloody stalemate on the battlefields of Europe. Yet the Spanish flu racked up a higher death toll than the war. Indeed, the widespread outbreak of the Spanish flu among troops on both sides helped end the fighting. Even the name of the illness was a misnomer connected to the war. Spain, a neutral country, was the only European government to allow early news reports about the disease to circulate. As a result, the public assumed the deadly flu was of Spanish origin. But the true source is still unclear.

The first reported cases of the Spanish flu arose in a military camp in Kansas in 1918. Troop movements around the United States and then overseas served to spread the deadly illness throughout the world. Eventually, the disease struck every continent on earth. Not even Pacific islanders or native peoples in remote areas of Alaska were spared.

Contagion in Crowded Conditions

Crowded conditions in tenements and military training camps caused the Spanish flu to spread swiftly. Unlike ordinary seasonal flu, which typically threatens the elderly and those with weak immune systems, the Spanish flu attacked healthy young people in large numbers. Beginning with chills and fever, it advanced rapidly to pneumonia. Patients could show the first signs of illness in the morning and be near death by nightfall. Lack of oxygen gave victims' skin a bluish tinge. Nurses like Lillian Clayton would check incoming patients for blackened feet, a sign of extremely poor oxygen supply in the blood and an indication that the victims were beyond help.

Health experts had few weapons to stop the Spanish flu from spreading. Knowledge about influenza and its causes was limited, and there were no vaccines or antibiotics for effective treatment. Many patients died not from the flu itself but from a secondary bacterial infection of the lungs. Doctors could offer little relief other than aspirin and hot compresses for the chest. Some prescribed

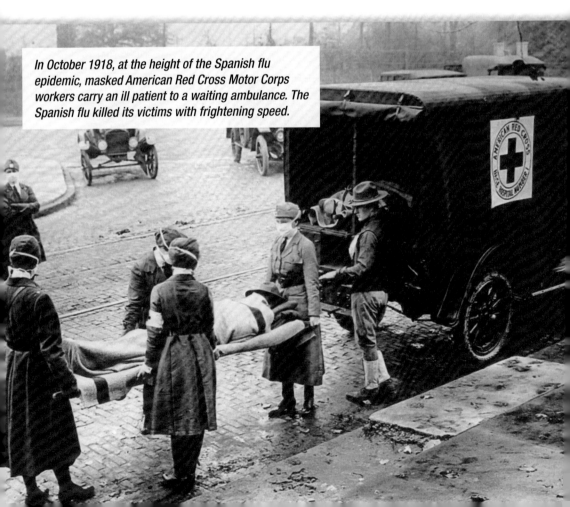

In October 1918, at the height of the Spanish flu epidemic, masked American Red Cross Motor Corps workers carry an ill patient to a waiting ambulance. The Spanish flu killed its victims with frightening speed.

hard liquor for their patients, while hucksters selling patent medicines laced with alcohol did a booming business. Civic leaders closed schools, churches, shops, and saloons; quarantined victims; and urged people with flu symptoms to wear a mask.

Lessons from the Outbreak

With the war's end in the fall of 1918, returning soldiers brought a second wave of even deadlier flu. The disease exploded into a worldwide catastrophe. War fatigue and economic collapse prevented nations from coordinating their health care efforts. In late 1919 and into 1920, a third wave struck nations in South Asia and East Asia especially hard. In India 18 million people died from flu-related illness, and Japan suffered huge losses.

> "The 1918 flu is still with us. . . . It never went away."[3]
>
> —Ann Reid, executive director of the National Center for Science Education

The Spanish flu is estimated to have killed about 2.7 percent of the world's population at the time. It laid bare the inadequacies of medical care in the United States and other countries. It also led to calls for more doctors, nurses, and hospitals, as well as increased government support for health care. Today traces of the Spanish flu virus continue to plague the world. "The 1918 flu is still with us, in that sense," says Ann Reid, executive director of the National Center for Science Education, who mapped the genome of the Spanish flu in the 1990s. "It never went away."[3]

CHAPTER ONE

A Pandemic Arises at the Great War's End

On Saturday, March 9, 1918, Private Albert Gitchell awoke feeling feverish and unable to perform his duties as company cook. Instead, Gitchell reported to the infirmary at Fort Riley's Camp Funston in north-central Kansas. The day dawned with high winds that promised to kick up a dust storm. Fires at the camp burned tons of manure from the company's horses and mules, turning the sky to yellow haze and making it difficult to breathe. Camp doctor Edward R. Schreiner found that Gitchell, one of fifty-six thousand soldiers stationed at the base, had a sore throat, headache, and high fever. Moreover, he was not alone. By noon more than one hundred of his fellow recruits were also complaining of flu symptoms. Within a month, those numbers had swelled to eleven hundred troops hospitalized. Thirty-eight victims died from pneumonia, their lungs choked with bloody fluid.

As the US Army rushed to prepare troops for warfare in Europe, barracks were crowded at military camps. Colds and flu spread like wildfire. However, the pathogen that arose at Fort Riley was no ordinary flu virus. It seemed to be highly contagious and especially deadly. The virus had already cropped up in nearby Haskell County. In January 1918 a local doctor named Loring Miner, fearing an outbreak of influenza, had alerted the US Public Health Service. After the Fort Riley cases appeared, physicians began to sound warnings in other military camps and crowded institutions around the country. In April five hundred prisoners fell ill at San Quentin State Prison in Northern California. By then there was no way for public health officials to gauge the spread among the civilian population.

Spreading the Illness to European Battlefields

At the time Americans were stoked with patriotic fervor. The United States had officially entered World War I—or the Great War, as it was then called—in April 1917. German submarine attacks on American merchant ships had inflicted large numbers of civilian casualties, inflaming passions in the United States. In a speech to Congress on April 2, 1917, President Woodrow Wilson had urged lawmakers to declare war on Germany, to win "the war to end all wars" and make the world "safe for democracy."[4] Howard Markel, a doctor and medical historian at the University of Michigan, notes that American society was immersed in the war effort. "We were getting involved in World War I and it was a very patriotic effort. You know, the war to end all wars," says Markel. "They were sending off young men in parades. Women were left behind and starting Red Cross chapters and making bandages and all sorts of things, sending the men off in a proper way."[5]

> "We were getting involved in World War I and it was a very patriotic effort.
> ... They were sending off young men in parades."[5]
>
> —Howard Markel, a doctor and medical historian at the University of Michigan

The spring of 1918 saw nearly one hundred thousand American soldiers and other personnel sailing to Europe each month. The arrival of US troops seemed to turn the tide in favor of the Allied powers, which included Great Britain and France. For war-weary Europeans, the war's end seemed finally in sight. However, a new enemy loomed on the horizon. American troop ships crossing the Atlantic were also carrying a deadly disease. It felled many troops before they reached the fighting. For

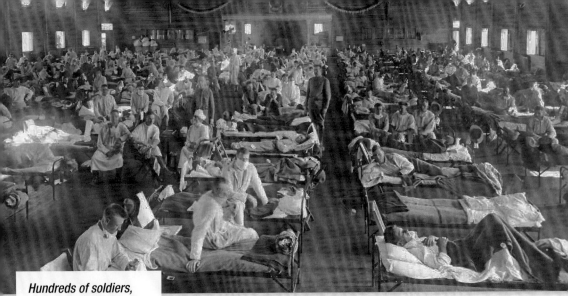

Hundreds of soldiers, sickened by Spanish flu, recuperate or receive care in the influenza ward at Fort Riley's Camp Funston. The flu virus that swept through the camp was highly contagious—and deadly.

example, thirty-six soldiers with the Fifteenth Cavalry Regiment caught the flu on their crossing to Europe. Six of them died.

Battlefield conditions in Europe were ideal for spreading the flu. The war had ground to a stalemate, with soldiers on each side huddled together in deep trenches protected by coils of barbed wire. Cold, damp, exhausted, and feverish to begin with, the troops could mount little resistance to the virus. The war, which had begun in July 1914, had already inflicted a horrific death toll in Europe. Now a raging flu outbreak threatened to add to the carnage. It would prove to be a more effective killer than all the machine guns, artillery shells, and poison gas on both sides combined.

Misnaming the Flu

By the late spring of 1918, soldiers and civilians in the warring nations were becoming sick with the flu. Their governments suppressed stories about the growing outbreak to lift morale and foil enemy propaganda. In the neutral country of Spain, however, news reports about the disease were not censored. Reporters were free to describe the flu outbreak plaguing Spanish cities and towns in detail. On May 22 the growing epidemic made headlines in Madrid's largest newspaper. Eventually, Alfonso XIII, the king of Spain, caught the disease, along with several members of his government. News reports from Madrid were headlined "Spanish King; Spanish Flu."

People around the world came to believe that the virus originated in Spain. The British press blamed the high winds and dry conditions in Spain for spreading dust filled with deadly microbes. Later research indicates that the flu probably reached Spain via migrant workers traveling by rail from France. Nonetheless, many newspapers began to call the disease the Spanish flu. "There was a very common habit, which has persisted to this day, of blaming an epidemic on one country or one group of people," says Markel. "It goes back centuries."[6]

Limited Knowledge About Influenza

The first wave of the Spanish flu was relatively mild compared to the later onslaught. Many referred to it as the three-day fever. Its symptoms—fever, body aches, a dry hacking cough, nausea, and diarrhea—were like those of a typical seasonal flu. Although data about public health at the time was limited, the mortality rate also seemed similar to normal flu viruses. Yet even this milder version of the Spanish flu was highly contagious and potentially lethal. Health officials struggled to control the outbreak. Lack of knowledge about influenza and its causes meant that attempts at treatment were ineffective and often misguided. Medical technology at the time offered few options to save the critically ill.

In 1918 scientists knew little about viruses in general. They did not know what they looked like, how to isolate them, nor how they behaved and mutated. In fact, doctors had yet to learn that influenza viruses even existed. Most health experts mistakenly blamed the Spanish flu outbreak on a bacterium called Pfeiffer's bacillus. "Clinicians and scientists of the time were grappling with many unknowns," says Terrence Tumpey, a microbiologist with the Centers for Disease Control and Prevention, "and what added to the confusion was the erroneous belief that the disease was caused by a bacterium. . . . It wasn't for another 30 years

13

that people would understand that the 1918 pandemic virus that infected 30% of the world's population was an influenza A (H1N1) virus."[7]

There were no vaccines for the flu and no antiviral drugs. Antibiotics had yet to be developed, with the discovery of penicillin a full decade away. Doctors had no diagnostic tests to determine whether a patient had a flu infection. Also, hospitals were understaffed, with many doctors and nurses having joined the war effort overseas. Most hospitals and clinics made do with few resources. There were no intensive care units and no mechanical ventilators to aid a patient's breathing. In many ways, physicians were stranded in the dark in their attempts to deal with the pandemic.

However, unknown to doctors at the time, one bright spot did emerge from the first months of the outbreak. According to recent research using military records, infections during the spring of

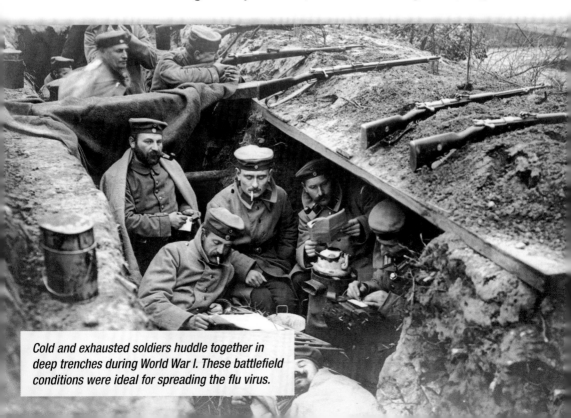

Cold and exhausted soldiers huddle together in deep trenches during World War I. These battlefield conditions were ideal for spreading the flu virus.

1918 acted like a vaccine. Most of those who got sick in the first wave of the Spanish flu developed an immunity. They proved to be 94 percent less likely to be stricken with the more severe second wave of illness. Researchers like Michael T. Osterholm, director of the University of Minnesota Center for Infectious Disease Research and Policy, believe this discovery about the 1918 flu could lead to rethinking policies about modern pandemics. "If we have wave one and it's relatively mild, and a number of people are exposed to that virus, that may actually be a very positive thing relative to a second wave in which the disease is much more severe," says Osterholm. "That could mean a lot of infection in a first wave is actually a good thing, with much of the world not having a vaccine."[8]

> "If we have wave one and it's relatively mild, and a number of people are exposed to that virus, that may actually be a very positive thing relative to a second wave in which the disease is much more severe."[8]
>
> —Michael T. Osterholm, director of the University of Minnesota Center for Infectious Disease Research and Policy

Fighting the Flu with Practical Measures

The first wave of the Spanish flu spread from army camps to civilian populations, mostly in the eastern United States. Troop movements by train accelerated the spread as soldiers made their way to embarkation ports on the East Coast. With few options for treatment of the sick, military officers turned to practical measures. They inspected bases and camps daily and placed suspected cases in isolation wards. Personnel with a temperature above 99°F (37.2°C) went to the base hospital. Camp buildings were cleaned and disinfected, tents and bedding aired out daily, and recovering patients kept in isolation for ten days. Some camps even imposed limits of five soldiers per tent to prevent spreading.

Those hospitalized with serious illness had to rely on the basics of nursing care. Military nurses could provide little more than fresh linens, cold compresses, sponge baths, water, soup, and medicines to relieve the pain. In the first wave, cases generally were resolved within three days, and deaths were infrequent. By late spring, the influenza seemed to have subsided in the United States. Local newspapers presented rosy reports about flu outbreaks, insisting that army doctors had the situation under control. Public concern remained focused on the war in Europe. Yet a darker chapter of the Spanish flu pandemic was just beginning.

A More Lethal Mutation

In the late spring of 1918, as large numbers of American troops sailed for France, they carried the Spanish flu virus with them. Experts estimate that three-quarters of French troops contracted the virus that spring, along with half of the British forces fighting in France. As soldiers deployed to new positions and moved back and forth from battlefield to cities and villages, the virus spread throughout Europe. "The rapid movement of soldiers around the globe was a major spreader of the disease," says James Harris, a historian at Ohio State University who studies both infectious disease and World War I. "The entire military industrial complex of moving lots of men and material in crowded conditions was certainly a huge contributing factor in the ways the pandemic spread."[9]

"The rapid movement of soldiers around the globe was a major spreader of the disease."[9]

—James Harris, a historian at Ohio State University who studies both infectious disease and World War I

Medical historians believe that the Spanish flu somehow mutated, or changed, into a much more virulent strain. The new version that emerged could kill a person within twenty-four hours after the first signs of infection. It was like no influenza that doctors had seen before. However, it did resemble the earlier strain in one important way: it was highly infectious. The virus infected a person's upper respiratory system, enabling the disease to be transmitted very easily by way of droplets from coughs and sneezes. Cramped quarters in barracks, bunkers, and trenches—not to mention crowded apartments for civilian families—ensured that the virus would spread unchecked. Crowding also meant

16

Debating the Origin of the Spanish Flu

Historians still debate where the so-called Spanish flu originated. Although most believe that it arose first in Kansas, many have revised their views of its origin. One theory speculates that the deadly disease came from China. Mark Humphries, a historian at Canada's Memorial University of Newfoundland, traces the source of the virus to an almost forgotten episode of World War I. In 1917 the Allies mobilized ninety-six thousand Chinese laborers to aid the war effort behind the lines on the western front. The workers traveled eastward across Canada in sealed train cars on their way to waiting ships. Humphries contends that these laborers spread the virus upon arrival in Europe.

Further research has found that a respiratory illness much like the Spanish flu hit northern China in November 1917. Medical records show that three thousand of the Chinese laborers aboard the Canadian trains wound up in medical quarantine with flu-like illness. Moreover, historians note that China's mortality rate from the Spanish flu was lower than that of other nations, indicating a special immunity among the population. These findings have convinced many experts. According to Lehigh University historian James Higgins, "This is about as close to a smoking gun as a historian is going to get."

Quoted in Dan Vergano, "1918 Flu Pandemic That Killed 50 Million Originated in China, Historians Say," *National Geographic*, January 24, 2014. www.nationalgeographic.com.

that infected persons got a larger dose of the virus, which made the symptoms worse. Moreover, soldiers were already weakened by fatigue, malnourishment, and physical injuries, making them more susceptible to illness. A deficiency in vitamin B, for example, has been found to increase death rates in other pandemics.

In 2005 American scientists were able to sequence the genetic code of the Spanish flu's deadly second-wave mutation. This enabled them to reconstruct the virus and study its effects on lab animals. They found that the mutated strain copied itself very rapidly. It set off an intense reaction from a patient's immune system. This reaction produced a so-called cytokine storm, in which white blood cells and inflammatory molecules flood a patient's system. Instead of fighting the infection, this overload of immune response further weakens the body, thereby increasing the susceptibility to secondary infections like pneumonia. The body essentially

A Cartoonist Saved from the Flu

In 1918 millions of young Americans were anxious to enlist in the military and fight the Germans overseas. Fears about the Spanish flu pandemic were brushed off as irrelevant to what really mattered. Walt, a seventeen-year-old high school student, was too young to sign up. But he drew patriotic cartoons and dreamed of joining the American Expeditionary Force like his two older brothers. Finally, in September 1918 Walt decided he could wait no longer. On his enlistment form, he changed his birth year to 1900 and was accepted for training at Camp Scott near Chicago.

When the virus struck the camp, Walt became desperately ill. Two of his friends went to the infirmary and died the next day. An ambulance driver offered to take young Walt to his home in Chicago. "You've got a better chance at home," he said. "If we take you to the hospital, you may never come out." Back in his own bedroom, Walt suffered delirium and high fever, but under his parents' care, he managed to pull through. He went on to pursue his dream of becoming a professional cartoonist. Ten years later, Walt Disney produced an animated cartoon featuring his most famous creation: Mickey Mouse.

Quoted in Jim Korkis, "How Young Walt Disney Almost Died During a Pandemic," Mouse Planet, April 8, 2020. www.mouseplanet.com.

drowns itself in its attempt to kill the virus. Scientists believe the cytokine storm might be the key to why healthy young adults died in such large numbers from the Spanish flu. Although a strong immune system usually would be beneficial in helping young adults shrug off the flu, in this case it made the infection even more severe. This also meant that children and older adults fared better against the Spanish flu—a reversal of what doctors expected in an influenza outbreak.

All viruses mutate. The fact that the Spanish flu virus mutated to become *more* lethal was unusual. If a virus is so deadly that it kills those it infects before they can spread the disease, then the virus might stop spreading and reproducing. The general rule is that viruses mutate into milder forms to ensure they continue to be transmissible, or able to spread. However, scientists disagree on this theory. "It's a bit of a lazy thing that we can sometimes trot out as virologists, that evolution would favor a virus becoming less pathogenic," says Jonathan Ball, a professor of virology at the University of Nottingham in the United Kingdom. "It's not always true—evolution can favor a virus that can persist and transmit more."[10]

A Virus Hiding in Plain Sight

As the first wave of flu cases began to wane in the spring of 1918, Americans focused on other concerns. They followed news reports about the bloody war in Europe, hopeful that America's entry would help bring the fighting to a close. They debated Prohibition, the constitutional ban on the production and sale of alcoholic beverages in the United States. They discussed the suffragist movement to extend voting rights to women. Meanwhile, the Spanish flu virus was hiding in plain sight, ready to reemerge in the fall.

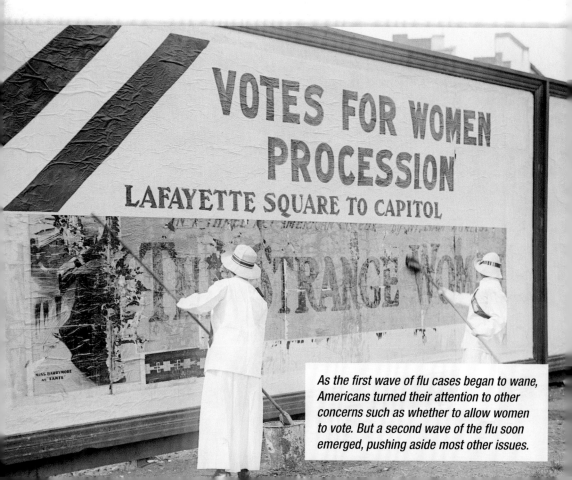

As the first wave of flu cases began to wane, Americans turned their attention to other concerns such as whether to allow women to vote. But a second wave of the flu soon emerged, pushing aside most other issues.

From its first appearance in Haskell County and Fort Riley in Kansas, the so-called Spanish flu had spread mostly among military personnel training for combat in Europe. The virus's first wave was less severe than later outbreaks and may have provided some immunity to those infected. Lack of knowledge about influenza and its causes limited what health officials could do to stop the disease from spreading. Crowded conditions in military camps, cities, and towns across the United States helped spread the highly infectious virus. Packed troop ships carried the virus to the battlefields of Europe, where a seemingly mutated version posed an even greater threat. Within months, the Spanish flu would explode with new ferocity in America and around the world.

CHAPTER TWO

A Deadly Second Wave

On October 8, 1918, Dr. John Anderson was taking his usual brisk walk down Riverside Avenue in downtown Spokane, Washington. Just ahead of him, a man paused to spit on the sidewalk, a not unusual practice at the time. Anderson was outraged, not just as a citizen but in his official capacity as chief public health officer of Spokane. With the Spanish flu sweeping the globe like a plague, health officials were at pains to make the public take it seriously. The local newspaper was not helping matters, having editorialized just recently that the seasonal influenza seemed milder than usual and declaring there was no cause for great alarm. One month before, Anderson himself had urged calm. He advised the people of Spokane to sneeze in their handkerchiefs, turn their heads when they coughed, and not worry about a widespread attack of the flu. Now, however, Anderson realized the true danger, and his patience was at an end. He ordered the man to use his own handkerchief to wipe the sidewalk clean.

The next day Anderson joined with seventeen local doctors to ban public gatherings in Spokane. Funerals and weddings were canceled, and schools, churches, theaters, and dance halls were closed until further notice. When it came to saving lives, Anderson did not hesitate to exert his authority—much like a military officer. "It is just as necessary to concentrate responsibility and authority in one man here as on the battlefield," Anderson said. "Perhaps more so, for the soldier fights a visible foe while the health authorities and the physician are combating an invisible enemy. All we see is results of the foe's strength."[11]

The Virus Reemerges

The more lethal Spanish flu that Anderson observed in Spokane had reached American shores by late August 1918. On August 27 a few sailors at Boston's Commonwealth Pier showed signs of infection. Two days later their number had risen to fifty-eight. By early September the virus had struck Camp Devens, an installation 40 miles (64 km) from Boston that housed fifty thousand men and a regional army hospital. Doctors there were astonished by the nature of the threat. They had never seen such severe respiratory illness. The first week of September, there were one hundred flu deaths each day at Camp Devens. By September 23 the number of cases had exploded to 10,500—more than in the nation's twenty-four other military camps combined.

Formerly healthy young soldiers were dropping dead within hours of first showing symptoms, while others struggled to survive for a few days. Patients with the usual flu symptoms of fever, chills, coughing, and nausea were rushed into isolation wards. Some already displayed deep brown spots on their cheeks, the telltale sign that suffocation had begun. Their lungs would begin to fill with a thick, bloody fluid. Lack of oxygen finally caused the victims' skin to turn a bluish purple—a condition called cyanosis—leading some to call the disease the Purple Death. As soldiers crowded into the infirmary, triage nurses would check patients' fingers and toes for the black or purplish color that indicated the case was hopeless. A doctor stationed at Camp Devens described the Spanish flu in a letter to a physician friend:

> These men start with what appears to be an attack of la grippe or influenza, and when brought to the hospital they very rapidly develop the most viscous type of pneumonia that has ever been seen. Two hours after admission they have the mahogany spots over the cheek bones, and a few hours later you can begin to see the cyanosis extending from their ears and spreading all over the face, until it is hard to distinguish the coloured men from the white. It is only a matter of a few hours then until death comes, and it is simply a struggle for air until they suffocate. It is horrible.[12]

Doctors at the time had no knowledge about the explosion of cytokines, the proteins that trigger inflammatory response, which were flooding their patients' lungs and causing them to drown

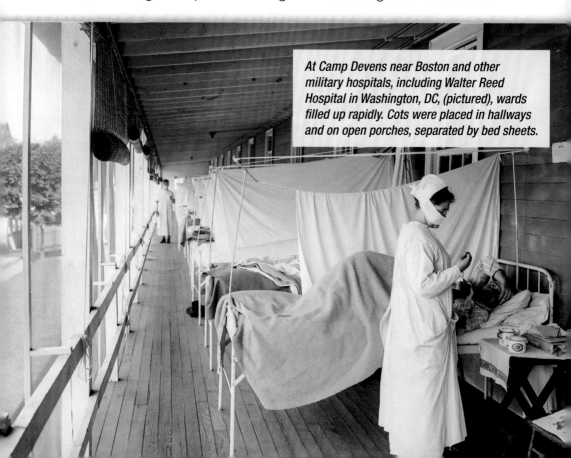

At Camp Devens near Boston and other military hospitals, including Walter Reed Hospital in Washington, DC, (pictured), wards filled up rapidly. Cots were placed in hallways and on open porches, separated by bed sheets.

in viscous fluids. However, some physicians did experiment with malarial drugs for treatment. These medications, which help curb inflammation, may have provided some benefit.

Surrounded by Death

Conditions grew worse at Camp Devens by late September. The hospital was overwhelmed with seriously ill patients, coughing and rasping. With sick wards crammed full, cots had to be lined up in hallways and on open porches. Soldiers shivering in blankets waited outside in the rain for a bed. Patients' gaunt blue faces announced their desperate state. The disease caused some to bleed from the nose, ears, and mouth. Visitors like Lieutenant Colonel William Henry Welch, an eminent physician and head of the National Academy of Sciences, were appalled at the chaos. To witness an autopsy and evaluate the disease, Welch had to step over piles of corpses in the Camp Devens morgue. Welch

Ending an Army Ban on Black Nurses

As the Spanish flu pandemic grew worse in the fall of 1918, army camps in the United States suffered a severe nursing shortage. Most qualified nurses were overseas caring for American soldiers in Europe. African American nurses were eager to fill the gap. However, the army's discriminatory policies did not allow them to serve in the US Army Nurse Corps. Black organizations and activists urged the American Red Cross and army officials to end the ban.

Finally, on December 1, 1918, three weeks after the war's end, the US Army Nurse Corps accepted eighteen African American nurses. They were assigned to Camp Sherman and Camp Grant in Ohio, facilities that housed large numbers of Black soldiers. There the nurses were able to treat both Black and White enlisted men with great energy and expertise. At Camp Sherman, when nurse Clara A. Rollins was scheduled for a transfer, the bedridden soldiers in her ward all signed a petition for her to stay. They called her "the major" and appreciated her dedication to providing the finest care. As Camp Sherman's chief nurse, Mary Roberts, recalled about her African American nurses, "They have done well with a vengeance."

Quoted in Valeri P., "These 18 Black Nurses Fought the 1918 Spanish Flu Pandemic and Paved the Way for Black Women in Nursing and Better Health in Black Communities," Urban Intellectuals, April 3, 2020. https://urban intellectuals.com.

looked on as the swollen lungs of a recently deceased soldier were removed. The lungs, filled with bloody, foamy fluid, struck Welch as evidence of some awful new plague. He immediately ordered the expansion of camp hospitals all over the country, as well as strict guidelines for quarantine.

Surrounded by death and in constant danger of infection themselves, medical personnel struggled to cope. One of the doctors at Camp Devens wrote:

> We have lost an outrageous number of Nurses and Drs., and the little town of Ayer [Massachusetts] is a sight. It takes special trains to carry away the dead. For several days there were no coffins and the bodies piled up something fierce; we used to go down to the morgue (which is just back of my ward) and look at the boys laid out in long rows. It beats any sight they ever had in France after a battle.[13]

The virus had begun to spread out of control, with more than fifty thousand people infected across Massachusetts by late September.

Similar scenes were starting to play out at other bases. Recruits were dying at an alarming rate. Moreover, deployment of nurses overseas meant that stateside military hospitals were badly understaffed. Josie Brown, a nurse at Naval Station Great Lakes near Chicago, admitted that the crush of new patients prevented any attempt at normal care. She noted that there was not enough time to take a patient's temperature or blood pressure. All she could offer as comfort was a small drink of whisky. Nurses like Brown also faced the constant risk of infection. When patients began to have nosebleeds from lung hemorrhages, blood could spew from their nostrils at any moment, sometimes shooting across the room. Amid the turmoil of the flu wards, medical workers had to fight back feelings of anxiety and helplessness.

Exploding Case Numbers in American Cities

By late September 1918 the Spanish flu had invaded American cities from coast to coast. Spreading from Camp Devens, the virus struck fifty thousand people in Boston and another twenty-five thousand in other areas of Massachusetts. By October 7 Boston had suffered 1,023 flu deaths. The city canceled war bond parades, sporting events, and church services. Schools closed, and the stock market opened only for half days. The flu pandemic soon took hold all over New England. To handle an overflow of patients, the Hartford Golf Club in Connecticut was pushed into service as an emergency hospital. Hundreds were dying in Hartford, New Haven, Bridgeport, and Waterbury. Vermont reported six thousand cases in the last week of September. A doctor in Portland, Maine, fearing an influx of flu cases from returning Canadian soldiers, begged the surgeon general to quarantine troop ships in Portland Harbor.

Case numbers also soared in New York City, Philadelphia, Chicago, San Francisco, and Seattle. Ships arriving at New York Harbor funneled flu patients, both sailors and civilians, straight to local hospitals. Daily cases rose from 999 on October 4 to nearly 5,000 on October 19. Death counts in New York City fluctuated between 400 and 500 each day. In Chicago as many as 60,000 people had fallen ill by October 5. Philadelphia recorded 700 deaths from the Spanish flu in one day. With so many young men falling sick nationwide, the army canceled a draft call for 142,000 men—this despite its desperate need for soldiers.

Like military physicians, doctors in urban hospitals were astonished at how quickly the disease could dispatch its victims. Some mistook it for a form of cholera or typhoid instead of influenza. Staggering numbers of deaths created new problems. Many cities were converting streetcars and delivery wagons into makeshift hearses to handle the growing number of corpses. Cemeteries posted jobs for extra grave diggers, since the usual crews were falling ill themselves or were afraid of catching the virus. Some states authorized prison inmates to dig graves on work release programs.

Flu Response Left to the States

As conditions across the United States worsened in the fall, the Wilson administration remained focused on fighting the war in Europe. To boost Americans' morale, Wilson intentionally hid the severity of the Spanish flu outbreak, even when hospitals and clinics became overwhelmed with the dead and dying. "Woodrow Wilson never made a public statement of any kind about the pandemic," says John M. Barry, a professor at the Tulane University

New York City's saloons, dance halls, and theaters were allowed to remain open as long as they improved their ventilation and banned smoking, coughing, and spitting. Posters like this one urged Americans to not spit because spitting was thought to help spread the flu virus.

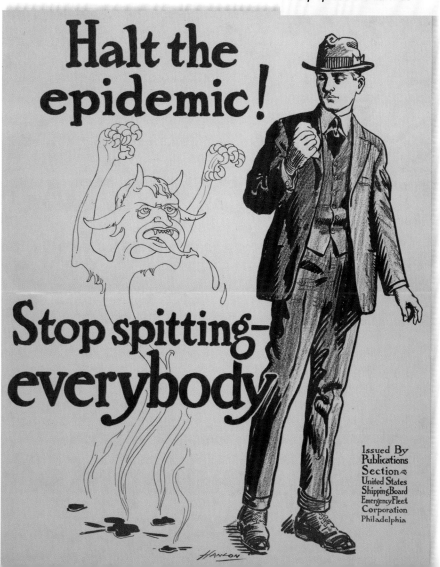

Halt the epidemic!

Stop spitting— everybody

Issued By
Publications
Section
United States
Shipping Board
Emergency Fleet
Corporation
Philadelphia

HANLON

School of Public Health and Tropical Medicine. "It was an indication of Wilson's intense focus on the war—that was all he cared about."[14] In addition, Wilson's administration clamped down on news reports about the pandemic and threatened to jail anyone whose speech might undermine the war effort. Expressing concern about the outbreak was condemned as unpatriotic. Such threats led newspapers to urge calm and to characterize the flu's impact as overblown. This in turn caused health experts at the state and local level to downplay the dangers—at least initially. However, as the deadly virus infected nearly one-quarter of all Americans, including some White House officials, it became impossible to hide the truth. Historians speculate that Wilson himself might have caught the disease in the autumn of 1918.

America's federalist system left the nation's response to the Spanish flu almost entirely to state and local governments. Governors, mayors, and health commissioners played a major role in shaping policies to stop the disease from spreading. Some moved swiftly to exert control. The governor of Alaska shut down its ports and enforced the closure with US Marshals. Officials in Ogden, Utah, sealed off the city completely, and citizens were required to show a doctor's note to get in or out. The mayor of Seattle closed all its churches and told the ministers who protested, "Religion that won't keep for two weeks, is not worth having."[15]

> "[President] Woodrow Wilson never made a public statement of any kind about the pandemic. It was an indication of Wilson's intense focus on the war—that was all he cared about."[14]
>
> —John M. Barry, a professor at the Tulane University School of Public Health and Tropical Medicine

Other officials, like New York City health commissioner Dr. Royal S. Copeland, sought a middle ground between widespread lockdowns and a business-as-usual approach that might endanger the population. On September 12, as flu cases began to rise, Copeland placed the entire Port of New York under quarantine. One week later, he invoked the city's sanitary code to force flu patients into isolation. "When cases develop in private houses or apartments they will be kept in strict quarantine there," Copeland told the *New York Times*. "When they develop in boardinghouses or tenements they will be promptly removed to city hospitals, and held under strict observation and treated there."[16]

Yet Copeland also insisted on keeping schools open, believing that children were better off in clean, well-ventilated classrooms than in cramped, dirty tenements. Only students who coughed or sneezed in class were sent home. Copeland also allowed most offices and stores to carry on, although with opening and closing times staggered to reduce crowding on public transportation. Saloons, dance halls, and theaters could remain open as long they improved their ventilation and banned all smoking, coughing, and spitting. Copeland's policies drew fire from those who wanted the city shut down for the

"When cases develop in private houses or apartments they will be kept in strict quarantine there. When they develop in boardinghouses or tenements they will be promptly removed to city hospitals."[16]

—Dr. Royal S. Copeland, New York City health commissioner

Overdosing on Aspirin

With so few options available for treating the Spanish flu, doctors turned to a relatively new wonder drug: aspirin. The US surgeon general recommended aspirin for treatment of flu symptoms. Versions of the drug had become widely available due to Bayer's recent loss of its exclusive patent. However, new manufacturers often failed to include warnings on aspirin packages about toxicity and proper use. Some medical historians now believe that overuse of aspirin may have added to the Spanish flu's death toll in the United States.

Medical experts at the time suggested doses of aspirin that today are considered extreme. The *Journal of the American Medical Association* advised that patients should receive 1,000 milligrams every three hours. This works out to nearly twenty-five standard tablets in twenty-four hours, or roughly twice the daily amount doctors today consider safe. Some researchers believe that heavy doses of aspirin could have contributed to bloody fluid in patients' lungs, the chief cause of death from the Spanish flu. As Peter A. Chyka, a professor of pharmacy at the University of Tennessee, notes, "There are things other than flu that can complicate a disease like this."

Quoted in Nicholas Bakalar, "In 1918 Pandemic, Another Possible Killer: Aspirin," *New York Times*, October 12, 2009. www.nytimes.com.

duration of the pandemic. However, New York City, with its per capita death rate of 452 deaths per 100,000, fared best of all other cities on the Eastern Seaboard.

Backlash Against Masking

With cases and deaths skyrocketing and no possibility of a vaccine, cities across America employed practical measures to control the Spanish flu. Governments isolated those with flu symptoms; banned public gatherings; mandated social distancing; closed shops, restaurants, bars, theaters, schools, and churches; and restricted use of public transportation. In many places, however, the most controversial laws involved wearing a mask.

Health officials promoted mask wearing as a simple step to avoid catching or spreading the virus. A cloth mask could protect its wearer and other people from airborne droplets produced by sneezing, coughing, spitting, or even talking. Since a person infected with the Spanish flu could be contagious for days before showing symptoms, experts recommended that everyone wear masks as a daily precaution. Several cities, including Sacramento and San Francisco, passed laws requiring masks to be worn on the street. One popular jingle urged people: "Obey the laws, and wear the gauze. Protect your jaws from septic paws."[17] Newspapers and magazines promoted masks for public health, showing how to make them and how to wear them properly. Most public service ads about masking addressed males, since females were thought less likely to need reminders. The Red Cross warned that any man, woman, or child refusing to wear a mask was a dangerous slacker. The campaign met with widespread success. Compliance with mask laws was generally high. Photographs of the period show army recruits, nurses, office workers, shopkeepers, spectators at sporting events, and ordinary pedestrians wearing cloth masks.

"Obey the laws, and wear the gauze. Protect your jaws from septic paws."[17]

—A popular jingle from 1918 about wearing masks for flu prevention

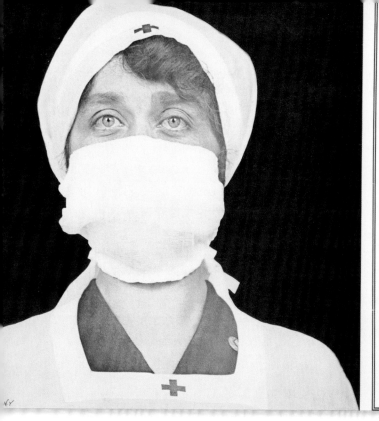

Health officials promoted mask wearing as a simple step to avoid catching or spreading the virus. A public service announcement offers prevention tips and shows a Red Cross nurse with a gauze mask over her nose and mouth.

Nonetheless, some Americans chafed at laws that required mask wearing. They attacked mask ordinances as a violation of civil rights. Some complained that masks were uncomfortable and unlikely to provide much protection. About the effectiveness of masks, they sometimes had a point. Detroit's health commissioner said that most homemade masks were too porous to provide genuine protection against the flu. In Phoenix and other cities, people began to cut holes in their masks for smoking, thus limiting their utility.

As the pandemic wore on, cities increased penalties for failing to wear masks in public. Violators were fined, jailed, and often listed by name in the newspaper. In Tucson, Arizona, a judge levied a ten-dollar fine on a person who pleaded that his mask was in the wash. In San Francisco an officer for the board of health shot a man who refused to don a mask. Two bystanders also were wounded in the incident.

Success and Failure Versus the Flu

Historians today note that cities' death rates from the Spanish flu depended on how prompt and aggressive they were in their response. For example, in late September 1918 Philadelphia, Pennsylvania, faced an outbreak from military personnel. Health officers knew that more than six hundred enlisted men in a camp just outside the city were showing flu symptoms. Forty-seven civilians had also been infected. Yet on September 28 public health director Wilmer Krusen refused to cancel an enormous Liberty Loan parade to promote the purchase of war bonds. Two hundred thousand people lined Broad Street in downtown Philadelphia. The tightly packed crowd cheered as troops in uniform, women's auxiliary groups, marching bands, military aircraft, and colorful floats filed past. The fallout from the event was predictable. Two days after the parade, Krusen delivered the bad news: the flu was tearing through the civilian population. Within three days, every bed in Philadelphia's thirty-one hospitals was occupied. On October 3 council members locked down the city. By October 12 more than forty-five hundred people in Philadelphia had died from the flu and related lung infections. Six weeks after the parade, twelve thousand were dead. Bodies were piled on the sidewalks due to overflow conditions at the morgues.

By contrast, officials in St. Louis, Missouri, were swift and decisive in their reaction to the virus. St. Louis saw its first cases of the Spanish flu arrive on October 5. Within two days, the city health commissioner, Dr. Max C. Starkloff, ordered shops, schools, saloons, and movie theaters to close. Weddings and funerals were canceled, and church services were suspended. In November, with the flu still rampant, Starkloff tightened the quarantine even further, shutting down banks and newspapers. Even coffin makers were ordered to stay home. As in other cities, only factories essential to wartime production remained open. Medical officers minded the factory floors, checking for coughs or sneezes. Although the Spanish flu killed nearly three thousand in St. Louis in the final months of 1918, the city's prompt action saved lives. St. Louis's death rate per one hundred thousand people was about half that of Philadelphia's.

In the fall of 1918, the deadly second wave of the Spanish flu hammered America. Spreading from military camps to cities and towns, the disease killed thousands of otherwise healthy young adults. State and city health officials across the nation led efforts to control the outbreak. Some imposed strict lockdowns and mandates for wearing masks, while others relied on fewer legal restrictions and more personal responsibility among citizens. Overall, the death counts in the United States proved catastrophic. In October 1918 alone, more than 195,000 people lost their lives to the Spanish flu. It remains the deadliest month in American history.

CHAPTER THREE

The Spanish Flu Becomes a Global Catastrophe

The British audience settling into their seats at the local movie house were about to get a jolt. It was January 1919, and the theater was showing, before the main picture, a short public service feature called *Dr. Wise on Influenza*. In the flickering black-and-white film, the bespectacled Dr. Wise is lecturing on the dangers of the Spanish flu. An ordinary worker is shown waking up feeling tired and feverish but then going to the office anyway. By not staying home, he spreads the flu to his fellow employees, who in turn pass it on to family members and friends. Then Dr. Wise reveals the film's true villain: wriggling bacteria viewed under a microscope, the apparent source of influenza. Dr. Wise promotes wearing masks of heavy gauze and frequent hand washing but warns that may not be enough to foil the tiny invaders. At any rate, the audience would not soon forget those pulsing microbes on the screen—the armies of a modern pandemic.

The film's glimpse of actual microbes was misleading. Influenza is not caused by bacteria, as shown in the film, but by a virus. Microscopes of the period were not powerful enough to view viruses. However, the film did break ground by focusing on the Spanish flu in the first place. British cinema had carefully avoided the subject, as did films from other European countries. "It's astonishing to think how invisible the first pandemic in the time of cinema is from the film record," says Bryony Dixon of the British Film Institute. "Apart from [*Dr. Wise on Influenza*], . . . the influenza pandemic of 1918/1919 doesn't appear in British film at all. There were no newsreel reports, and no fiction films were made that even mentioned the three waves of the pandemic."[18]

Refusal to Order Quarantines

British media mostly stayed mum about the Spanish flu. It went unmentioned in Parliament for months. Yet the mutated virus raged throughout Europe in the fall of 1918, adding to the Continent's misery from the war. In September British soldiers infected with the virus returned home after years in the trenches of northern France. They complained of la grippe (the European shorthand for colds and flu), with symptoms of headache, sore throat, and loss of appetite. The flu spread like wildfire in England, infecting even David Lloyd George, the prime minister and head of the wartime coalition government. The fifty-five-year-old Lloyd George contracted the disease after accepting an honorary award outdoors amid pouring rain and congratulatory handshakes in Manchester. For eleven days, the prime minister remained stuck in Manchester, anchored to a hospital bed set up in the local town hall. To aid the war effort, news reporters kept Lloyd George's condition under wraps and rarely mentioned the Spanish flu at all. When the prime minister was finally able to travel, he wore a respirator to aid his damaged lungs.

As in the United States, most British victims of the flu were healthy young adults aged twenty to thirty, with children and the elderly much less susceptible. This meant that workers in munitions factories across England—the factories that were running

The Impact on Young Women

The Spanish flu's devastating effect on males in their twenties and thirties is well documented. Yet the virus could be lethal to young women as well. British novelist Anthony Burgess describes a terrible scene from when he was two years old: "In early 1919 my father, not yet demobilized, came on one of his regular, probably irregular, furloughs to Carisbrook Street to find both my mother and sister dead. The Spanish Influenza had struck. . . . I apparently was chuckling in my cot while my mother and sister lay dead on a bed in the same room."

Burgess's mother was young and healthy when she succumbed to the disease. Children of parents who died from the flu were fortunate to survive themselves. (Burgess's four-year-old sister did not.) The Spanish flu also took a heavy toll on pregnant women. Those in their last trimester of pregnancy were five to nine times more likely to die of flu-related illness than nonpregnant women who were infected. Not surprisingly, the disease also resulted in many miscarriages.

Anthony Burgess, *Little Wilson and Big God.* London: Heinemann, 1987, p. 18.

overtime to supply war materials—were especially prone to infection. With conditions so cramped on the factory floor, one case could quickly proliferate into twenty, then one hundred, then five hundred. Nonetheless, by order of Arthur Newsholme, the chief medical officer of the Local Government Board, British officials took few actions to address the threat of flu. (Health care in Britain at the time was the responsibility of local authorities.) In July 1918, Newsholme had issued a public notice for citizens to isolate themselves if sick and to avoid large groups, but now he decided that the war effort outweighed all other considerations. He made sure that factories remained open with no exceptions, as well as almost all other offices, shops, and businesses. He also refused to order quarantines for people showing flu symptoms. Among the British, Newsholme became known for his stiff-upper-lip approach to serious hardship. "There are national circumstances in which the major duty is to 'carry on,'" he said, "even when risk to health and life is involved."[19] And while many British citizens appreciated Newsholme's spirit, his policies led to a disastrous number of lives lost. In 1918, for the first time since government record keeping had begun in 1837, Britain's death rate exceeded its birth rate.

Success with Stronger Measures

Historians note that there were alternatives to Newsholme's lax program. In Manchester, where the prime minister had been laid up for nearly two weeks, the city's medical officer took stronger measures against the virus, with great success. James Niven, a Scottish doctor, perceived at once that the flu would spread rapidly on the crowded sidewalks of his industrial city. He advised schools, movie theaters, restaurants, and offices to close at once. He urged people to wear masks and to maintain several feet of separation from others—or what is now called social distancing.

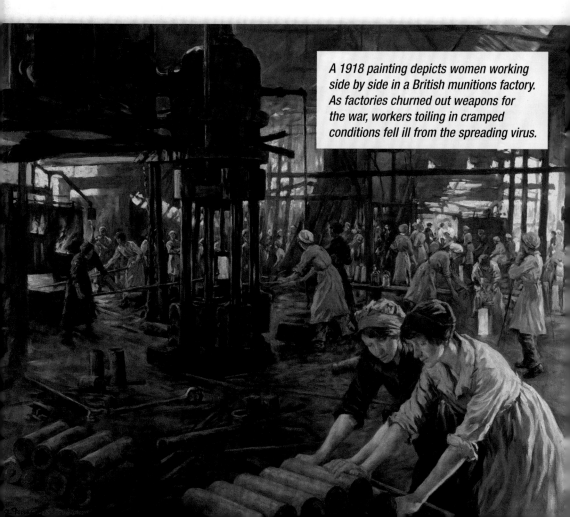

A 1918 painting depicts women working side by side in a British munitions factory. As factories churned out weapons for the war, workers toiling in cramped conditions fell ill from the spreading virus.

He hammered home the need for personal hygiene and warned against sharing towels, soap, and washbasins. People who came down with the virus faced immediate quarantine.

Niven also wrote a column for the *Manchester Guardian* outlining the best precautions against the flu. "On no account join assemblages of people for at least 10 days after the beginning of the attack," he advised readers who came down with flu symptoms, "and in severe cases . . . remain away from work for at least three weeks."[20] Under Niven, Manchester achieved one of the lowest death rates from the flu in the entire country. By late 1918 Newsholme had seen the benefits of Niven's approach. In response, he arranged to educate the British public in a novel way—with the film *Dr. Wise on Influenza*.

A Society Upended by the Flu

As the grueling war in Europe ground to a halt, British society found itself nearly upended by the Spanish flu. London seemed as helpless in confronting the pandemic as any rural village. The war had drained the nation's finances and killed more than seven hundred thousand enlisted men, or 11 percent of those in uniform. Now the deadly virus was placing a huge burden on public services that were already faltering. Hospitals were swamped with new patients, and doctors and nurses were strained to the breaking point. Medical schools canceled classes for third- and fourth-year students, recruiting them instead to assist in flu wards. Cities took to spraying streets with disinfectant in a desperate attempt to subdue the outbreak. People shared theories about how to escape the disease, including eating porridge, drinking cocoa, brushing one's teeth, taking long walks—women at the War Department took a fifteen-minute stroll in the fresh air each morning—and even smoking more cigarettes to protect the lungs. Companies took

Ancient Herbal Treatments in China

While Europe and the United States suffered high death rates from the second wave of the Spanish flu, China managed to keep mortality rates fairly low. Researchers who believe the Spanish flu originated in China also theorize that the Chinese people had some level of immunity to the virus. That would explain why many places in China, such as Shanghai and Hong Kong, seemed to have more success fending off the disease.

Some Chinese experts also link the nation's lower death rates to ancient herbal medicines and natural methods of prevention. Instead of turning to Western medicine, the Chinese relied on treatments that went back hundreds and even thousands of years. For example, the local government of Chengde County in Hebei Province announced unusual measures to address the pandemic. Villagers were told that "houses should be sprayed with limewater or lime powder, and rhubarb . . . should be burned to disinfect the air." They were urged to "drink more soup prepared with powdered mung bean and rock sugar, several times a day." The program proved successful, since more than 97 percent of local people who contracted the flu were able to recover—a much higher rate than in places like San Francisco.

Quoted in K.F. Cheng and P.C. Leung, "What Happened in China During the 1918 Influenza Pandemic?," Science-Direct, 2007. www.sciencedirect.com.

advantage of the flu panic to promote their products as sources of flu resistance. Sanatogen, a tonic made mostly of milk protein, was advertised as a boost to the nervous system. Oxo, a beef broth made from slaughterhouse scraps, claimed to fight off infection. As one ad put it, "A cupful of OXO two or three times a day will prove an immense service as a protective measure. . . . One's aim must be the maintenance of strength."[21]

Disposing of the dead presented more signs of societal breakdown. The military draft had left funeral parlors and cemeteries severely understaffed across Great Britain. Grave diggers and undertakers found themselves in great demand. Lack of both horses and quality feed meant that few wagons were available to transport the deceased. In Sunderland, a port city in northeastern England, more than two hundred bodies lay unburied for more than a week.

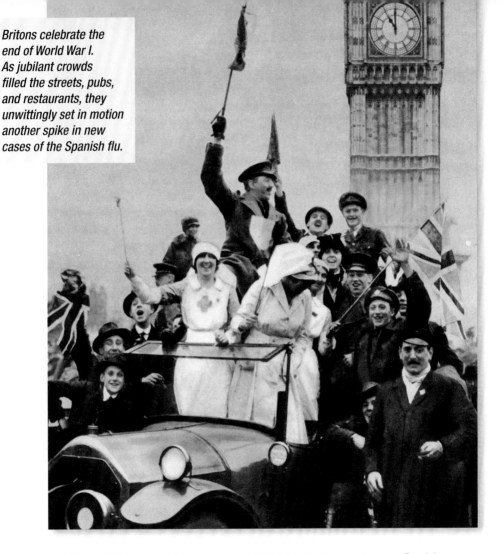

Britons celebrate the end of World War I. As jubilant crowds filled the streets, pubs, and restaurants, they unwittingly set in motion another spike in new cases of the Spanish flu.

That fall even a joyous event led to further misery. On November 11 the Great War ended in an armistice, or an agreement by both sides to stop fighting. Delirious crowds poured into the streets in London and other large cities. Brass bands played, and pubs and restaurants filled with happy patrons for the first time in weeks. Inevitably, the mass celebrations brought another spike in new cases of the Spanish flu. Some soldiers returned home only to find that the flu had struck their families. According to Hannah Mawdsley, a historian at Queen Mary University of London, "There are heartrending accounts of soldiers who had survived four years of war, only to be heading home and receiving the news their wives or family members had died before they could get back."[22]

The pandemic in Great Britain continued for several more months, coming to an end in the summer of 1919. Overall, about 228,000 British people died from the disease.

A Disastrous Outbreak in India

By the war's end, the Spanish flu had spread to every corner of the world. An estimated one-third of the world's population was eventually infected. At the height of the pandemic, Paris suffered more than twelve hundred flu deaths each week. Hundreds were dying each day throughout Italy and Spain. The disease killed four hundred thousand German civilians in one year. Homebound British Commonwealth and colonial troops also carried the disease to far outposts in India, Australia, New Zealand, and African nations. The death count in Europe, while considerable, was dwarfed by numbers in Asia and Africa.

The virus proved to be especially lethal in British India. In late May 1918, infected Bengal troops returning to India from the trenches of the Great War brought the Spanish flu with them. Three months later case numbers began to soar in the capital city of Bombay (now called Mumbai). More than 290 people had died there by September 19. The virus swept through India along trade lines and postal routes, striking cities and villages along the way. Indian newspaper reports described 150 to 200 bodies a day being fed into furnaces for cremation. Burial grounds became overrun with corpses. Jackals waited until nightfall to feast on the dead.

The nation's British rulers dwelt in spacious estates that were barely touched by the outbreak. Most of their letters to London failed to mention any problems with influenza. By contrast, the common people of India, living in crowded, dirty neighborhoods, could not avoid the catastrophe. As the sanitary commissioner of

"There are heartrending accounts of soldiers who had survived four years of war, only to be heading home and receiving the news their wives or family members had died before they could get back."[22]

—Hannah Mawdsley, a historian at Queen Mary University of London

Punjab noted, "The streets and lanes of cities were littered with dead and dying people . . . nearly every household was lamenting a death, and everywhere terror and confusion reigned."[23]

Although the entire subcontinent of India fell prey to the disease, the northern and western areas were especially hard hit, with 4.5 percent to 6 percent of their total populations killed. Deaths were divided along class lines. Lower-caste Indians in Bombay were nearly eight times more likely to die from the flu than the British colonials. In addition, they suffered from food shortages blamed on British agricultural reforms. From 1918 to 1920, about 18 million Indians died from the Spanish flu or related illness, equal to the total death toll of World War I. The pandemic also hastened social and political change in India. Resentful of British rule, India's people were well aware of the disparities in health outcomes. "There is a good case to be made that the devastation wrought by the disease exacerbated social tensions in India," says science journalist Laura Spinney, "contributing to an eruption of violence and significantly strengthening the independence movement."[24]

> "There is a good case to be made that the devastation wrought by the disease exacerbated social tensions in India, contributing to an eruption of violence and significantly strengthening the independence movement."[24]
>
> —Laura Spinney, a British science journalist and author

The Value of Quarantines

British Commonwealth ships also spread the contagion to New Zealand, Australia, and the Pacific islands. Native islanders in Fiji, Tonga, Tahiti, and Nauru fell victim to the crew members' more virulent flu in October and November 1918. Like indigenous peoples elsewhere, such as the Inuit in Alaska, Pacific islanders seemed to lack natural defenses against the virus. At the same time, Western Samoa and American Samoa, in their starkly different responses to the virus, offered a prime example of the value of quarantines.

The two Samoas shared the same language and culture and enjoyed many blood ties among families. However, they diverged

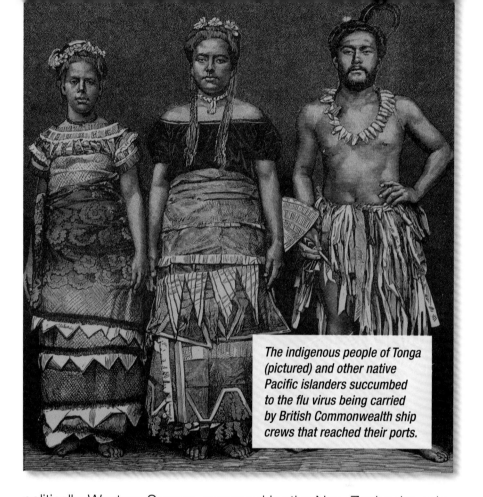

The indigenous people of Tonga (pictured) and other native Pacific islanders succumbed to the flu virus being carried by British Commonwealth ship crews that reached their ports.

politically. Western Samoa, governed by the New Zealander colonel Robert Logan, was still bound to colonialism and arbitrary rule. Logan administered the two large islands that make up Western Samoa with little thought about the interests of the native inhabitants. On November 7, when the New Zealand passenger and cargo ship *Talune* arrived in Western Samoa on its regular Pacific tour, its crew members were showing symptoms of the Spanish flu. Although other ports on the route had forbidden the crew to leave the ship, Western Samoan officials let sick passengers and crew members come ashore. Illness spread rapidly across the islands. Weeks later, 22 percent of the people on both Western Samoan islands had lost their lives to the virus. The arrival of four physicians from Australia in December came too late to stave off disaster.

By contrast, US Navy commander John Martin Poyer, American Samoa's governor, quarantined all ships that arrived in Pago

Pago Harbor, the largest port among the islands. This included the *Talune*, which docked in Pago Pago four days before its fateful trip to Western Samoa. Poyer placed passengers showing symptoms under house arrest. He also assigned Samoans and Whites to separate clinics, a move based partially on the islands' existing racial boundaries and partially on US Navy policy. This had the hidden benefit of distancing the more vulnerable native peoples from the deadly virus.

In making these decisions, Poyer relied on input from the local Samoan chiefs, or *matais*. The *matais* supported the strict quarantines as best for the welfare of their own people. Poyer even deputized Samoan youths to patrol the shores in small boats to foil anyone trying to evade the quarantine. As a result, not a single case of the Spanish flu broke out in American Samoa. As a tribute to the Samoans' cooperation, Poyer recommended the three district chiefs of the islands for presidential medals. As Poyer wrote, "The fact that no case of influenza broke out in our islands . . . [is due] in no small measure, to the influence exerted over the natives by these chiefs."[25]

Adding to the War's Misery

The Spanish flu outbreak in the fall of 1918 added to Europe's misery from the war. Civilians who were already struggling with food shortages and job losses fell to the virus in huge numbers. Health officials in Great Britain generally refused to order quarantines for fear of damaging the war effort. Such policies doubtless cost lives and wrecked families. Despite the Spanish flu's deadly effects, the disease was scarcely mentioned by European governments and media intent on preserving wartime morale.

Eventually the virus spread around the world. Its killing force was magnified in colonial outposts such as British-ruled India, where ordinary people lived in cramped conditions that were ideal for spreading the flu. The disease presented a special threat to indigenous peoples of the East and West. By war's end, it was obvious that the Spanish flu would have long-term impacts on societies the world over.

CHAPTER FOUR

The End and Aftereffects

The first reports of the Spanish flu in Japan concerned a Japanese obsession: sumo wrestling. In April 1918 a group of the enormous wrestlers began to display flu symptoms while on tour in Taiwan. Alarmingly, three of the best-known grapplers became seriously ill and died before they could return home. Among them was the great Masagoishi, widely regarded as the next superstar of sumo. With the virus spreading in Japan, officials canceled a major sumo tournament scheduled for the summer. The high-profile deaths led the Japanese to label the Spanish flu as the *sumo kaze*, or "sumo cold."

Another Japanese nickname for the virus was *guntai byo*, or "the military disease." This referred to 150 sailors who contracted the flu aboard the warship *Shubo* docked at the Yokosuka naval base. By the fall Japan's first wave of the Spanish flu was paralyzing the nation. Female textile workers in Ogaki were laid low with high fevers and sudden nosebleeds. More than one-fifth of the drivers for Osaka's electric railways fell ill, interrupting rail service for days. Bodies were piling up in hospitals and crematoriums. Death announcements could not be sent by telegram because so many operators were stricken with the flu. But the worst was still ahead.

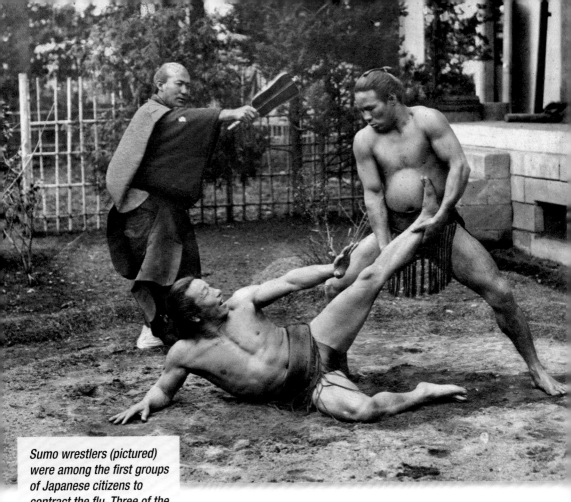

Sumo wrestlers (pictured) were among the first groups of Japanese citizens to contract the flu. Three of the best-known wrestlers died from the flu before they could return home from events being held in Taiwan.

The Third Wave Strikes

Japan was among the last countries in the world to battle the Spanish flu, along with nations in the Southern Hemisphere such as Brazil, Australia, and many African nations. Although the third wave that struck the West in 1919 was relatively mild, it presented a much graver threat in Japan. During this final outbreak, Japanese health officials released five recommendations to survive the pandemic: stay away from the sick, avoid crowds, wear a mask in public (a common Japanese response to contagions), gargle regularly, and provide extra care for the very old and very young. The government took a proactive approach, communicating with the people through newspaper notices, posters on the street, and leaflets passed out in schools. Geoffrey Rice, a historian based in

New Zealand, believes the Japanese approach offers a valuable lesson for dealing with a pandemic: "The main lesson from the 1918 flu in Japan . . . was that the response had to be a widely based community effort. The crucial response was at the street and community level. We cannot hope to know everyone on our street, but we should at least know those on either side [of us]. Assistance can then overlap down a street, like the overlapping tiles on the roof of a temple."[26]

Even with the public advisories, the disease raged throughout Japan. Young adults were losing their lives at an astounding rate. About 20 percent of those infected were dying of the flu, an unheard-of percentage. Entire villages were swept away by the virus. With no effective treatments available, some people took refuge in bizarre cures, such as a medication made of ground-up earthworms. Others relied on local herbal remedies and lots of green tea.

Newspapers in Tokyo and other major cities ran daily reports on the explosion of fatalities. The obituaries, framed in thick black borders, went on for pages. The Japanese called this period from mid-January to early February 1920 simply Three Weeks of Hell. By the end of the pandemic in Japan, more than 450,000 people had perished from the flu and related cases of pneumonia. An estimated 200,000 more died in Korea and Taiwan, which Japan administered as colonies.

> "The main lesson from the 1918 flu in Japan . . . was that the response had to be a widely based community effort. The crucial response was at the street and community level."[26]
>
> —Geoffrey Rice, a historian based in New Zealand

A Colonial Disaster in Africa

In East Africa the Spanish flu pandemic seemed to be fueled by the British colonial system. The virus first arrived in the port of Mombasa in Kenya via shipping from British-controlled Bombay. Having avoided the first, milder round of influenza, Africans in Kenya had no immunity to protect themselves from the deadliest effects of this later wave. Serving as a trading center for British war supplies and other goods, Mombasa distributed the virus along with endless loads of cargo. By October 1918 railway connections to the interior had delivered infected passengers all along the East African trade routes.

Colonial officials scrambled to head off the pandemic. They posted guidelines for medical personnel to avoid transmission, including washing their hands and practicing social distancing. Doctors were also urged to take quinine, an antimalarial drug, three times a day. Native Kenyans, by contrast, were told at first to nurse their sick at home, take a teaspoon of paraffin oil three times a day, and follow a diet high in calcium and starch. Infection among the locals resulted in lost jobs and forfeited salaries, preventing families from buying food and other necessary items. Subsistence farmers who managed to survive the virus were still likely to lose their crops, which were also a vital food source for

Black October in South Africa

Among African nations, South Africa suffered the worst losses from the Spanish flu. It was one of the five hardest-hit areas in the world. More than three hundred thousand South Africans, or 6 percent of the country's population, died of the flu and its complications in six weeks. As one doctor admitted in the *South African Medical Record* of January 1919, "It has truly been an irreparable calamity which has fallen on South Africa."

Mistakes compounded the disease's threat. In September 1918 two troop ships brought more than two thousand Black South African Native Labour Corps soldiers back to South Africa from the flu-ridden battlefields of Europe. Despite signs of flu among some of the soldiers, the corps' medical officer made only quick examinations of the sick men, and quarantines were not rigidly enforced. Three days after their arrival, all the soldiers were permitted to go home. Traveling by rail to every corner of the country, they spread the virus first to stations along the way, then to families and friends in their home villages. Within a few weeks, the disease was raging throughout South Africa. As one magazine described the outbreak dubbed Black October, "[It was] allowed to run everywhere at once, like spilt quicksilver."

Quoted in Howard Phillips, "South Africa Bungled the Spanish Flu in 1918. History Mustn't Repeat Itself for COVID-19," The Conversation, March 10, 2020. www.theconversation.

their villages. When British clinics were overrun with new cases, panicked health care workers passed out placebo pills, or fake sugar pills, to pacify the locals. At the same time, most Kenyans with flu symptoms ignored quarantine orders and returned to their villages, helping spread the disease.

Within nine months of the flu's arrival, 150,000 Kenyans were dead, representing 4 to 6 percent of the total population. Unlike most outbreaks in the world, African deaths followed a pattern more typical of ordinary influenza, with victims concentrated among the aged. "Death occurred mostly among the old men and women," wrote a British assistant district commissioner, "and judging from the number of elders of council reported to have died must have run into hundreds."[27] Another district official blamed the deaths on overcrowding and food shortages. Certainly, malnutrition played its part in the catastrophe. Few among the colonial authorities recognized the level of smoldering anger among Kenyans over the British response to the pandemic.

> "Death occurred mostly among the old men and women, and judging from the number of elders of council reported to have died must have run into hundreds."[27]
>
> —A British assistant district commissioner in Kenya

A New Year Filled with Hope

As the calendar flipped to January 1, 1919, people around the world sought to banish thoughts of war and disease. Americans threw themselves into wild celebrations, from society balls in New York City's Manhattan to neighborhood parties in the outer boroughs. With Prohibition rumored to be in the works, many toasted the new year with alcoholic drinks that might soon be illegal. Even with the war over, newspapers continued mostly to avoid the subject of the Spanish flu. Obituaries of young adults, of which there were still too many, generally did not include the cause of death, leading readers to assume the victims died of the flu. Health experts stressed that the pandemic was far from over. Dr. Royal Copeland, New York City's beleaguered commissioner of health, continued to warn people about spreading the virus: "The person who coughs or sneezes discharges a spray more deadly than bullets or poison gas, unless the mouth and nose are covered by a handkerchief."[28] But most people were ready to throw caution to the wind. The Spanish flu would persist until the summer, although death totals steadily diminished.

Seeking the Virus in a Lost Village

The disease by then had reached nearly every corner of the world, including the most remote enclaves of indigenous people. One of these was the tiny village of Brevig Mission, on the Seward Peninsula in northern Alaska. Whether through contact with traders pulled by dog teams or with a postal delivery agent, the Spanish flu had finally come to Brevig Mission in the fall of 1918. Most of the village's eighty inhabitants were native Inuit accustomed to the harsh realities of the Alaskan frontier. But like indigenous peoples elsewhere in the world, they lacked immune defenses against the disease. In a five-day span from November 15 to 20, seventy-two of the villagers died from the flu.

The local government created a mass grave site on a hill alongside the village. Gold miners from Nome were hired to gouge a hole in the permafrost wide and deep enough to hold seventy-two bodies. Small white crosses were set in place to commemorate the victims and honor a small community that had nearly been wiped away. Chances were, the graves would be forgotten over time.

But fate intervened in the person of Johan Hultin, a microbiology student from Sweden. Hultin was obsessed with recovering the deadly Spanish flu virus—what he called "the most lethal organism in the history of man."[29] A virologist friend suggested that the way to recover the virus was to find bodies of flu victims that had been buried—and preserved—in frozen permafrost. On a trip to Fairbanks, Alaska, in 1949, Hultin managed to obtain records from a Lutheran church covering Alaskan communities in 1918. The records specified how villagers had died and where

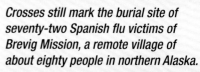
Crosses still mark the burial site of seventy-two Spanish flu victims of Brevig Mission, a remote village of about eighty people in northern Alaska.

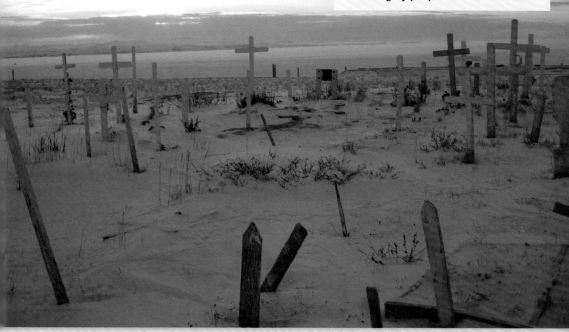

they were buried. Hultin checked the records of flu deaths against a permafrost map to find the best possibility for his research project: the village of Brevig Mission.

In 1951 he flew in to discuss his plan with village elders. With their permission, Hultin and three scientist friends set aside the remaining white crosses and opened the mass grave. Inside, the bodies had been sufficiently preserved by the frozen soil. Hultin took lung tissue from four bodies and then helped close the grave. Returning to his lab in Iowa, he tried a number of different ways to revive the Spanish flu virus. Nothing worked, and he abandoned the project.

Bringing the Virus Back to Life

Forty-six years later, Hultin, now age seventy-one, got a second chance to see his goal realized. In the journal *Science*, he read about a scientist named Jeffery Taubenberger, whose team at the National Institute of Allergy and Infectious Diseases was working on isolating genetic material from viruses. His latest effort involved removing samples from the tissue of two young soldiers who fell victim to the Spanish flu in 1918. Taubenberger's problem was that his samples were too small, about the size of a thumbnail. Intrigued, Hultin wrote to say he knew where larger samples could be found.

In August 1997 Hultin returned to Brevig Mission, which was now a town of four hundred. He obtained the elders' permission once more and reopened the mass grave. Seven feet (2.1 m) down, he discovered the well-preserved body of a large woman. Fatty tissue and the permafrost had protected the lungs from decay. Eight years later, using a sample from the woman's lungs, Taubenberger and his team were able to reconstruct a live version of the virus genetically. The team took extraordinary safety measures to avoid any chance of the potentially lethal virus escaping. They discovered that it had originally come from bird viruses and had adapted itself to infect people.

The Spanish Flu and Women's Suffrage

The Spanish flu disproportionately killed males the world over. At the same time, its ravages and disruptions provided new opportunities for females. In the United States, with thousands of young men sailing overseas to fight or battling the disease at home, labor shortages threatened to slow the war effort. Women were able to join the workforce and demonstrate their abilities like never before. As President Woodrow Wilson declared in a September 1918 speech to the Senate on women's suffrage: "This war could not have been fought . . . if it had not been for the services of the women—services rendered in every sphere."

Their expanded role changed attitudes about women's proper place in society. The so-called suffragettes found new acceptance for the idea of women's equality. Campaigning amid the war and pandemic, they stressed how women—whether as nurses at the front or factory workers at home—were also making sacrifices for their country. According to historian Allison K. Lange, "It was assumed that women would do this [nursing] work and risk their lives to be caregivers." A grateful nation rewarded their contributions. In 1920 the states ratified the Nineteenth Amendment, giving women the right to vote.

Quoted in Susin Haynes, "'Persevere Through the Highs and Lows.' What We Can Still Learn from the Suffragists Who Fought for the Right to Vote During the 1918 Flu Pandemic," *Time*, June 3, 2020. www.time.com.

Taubenberger and his team's *Jurassic Park*–style experiment continues to pay dividends. It has increased knowledge of how viruses, including the one that causes COVID-19, mutate from animal sources to human. According to Douglas Jordan, a health communications specialist with the Centers for Disease Control and Prevention, "The 1918 virus was special—a uniquely deadly product of nature, evolution and the intermingling of people and animals."[30]

Impact on Health Care in the Modern World

There are many reasons that the Spanish flu struck the world of 1918 with such force. The virus was especially contagious and lethal. Medical knowledge was limited, especially where viruses were concerned. A catastrophic war was going on, creating circumstances that only helped the disease to spread. In cities and towns, many people lived in crowded, unsanitary conditions without enough food. Large populations were ruled by colonial governments that rarely acted in their best interests. Yet in many ways the Spanish flu pandemic has affected the modern world just as much.

Failure to control the flu's spread caused people in many countries to push for better health care solutions. Physicians at the time were either self-employed or relied on funding from charities or religious groups. When the flu struck, many people barely had access to a doctor's care. Increasing numbers of people decided that governments bore responsibility for the lackluster response. There were growing calls for socialized medicine, which meant health care provided by the government free of charge for every citizen, regardless of status or means. Soviet Russia created a centralized system of health care, funding it with state-sponsored insurance. Nations of western Europe fashioned similar systems. The United States set up private health insurance

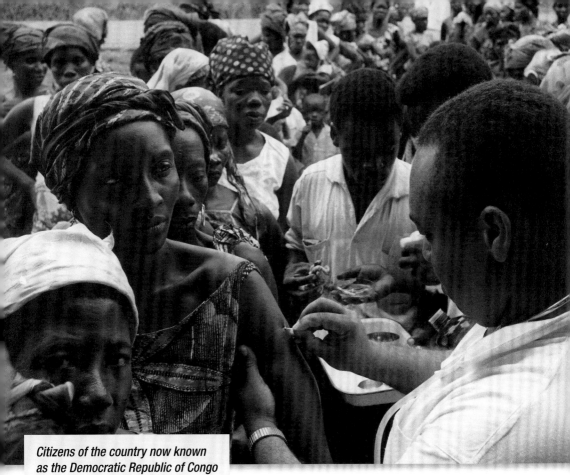

Citizens of the country now known as the Democratic Republic of Congo are vaccinated against smallpox in 1963. The clinic doing this work was run by the World Health Organization, which was created in response to the Spanish flu pandemic.

provided through employers, not the government. Each model sought to consolidate health care for the greatest possible benefit.

After the Spanish flu pandemic, epidemiology became a cornerstone of public health. Experts began to study the causes of infectious disease, as well as patterns of infection. Health officials worldwide realized that outbreaks of infectious disease do not recognize borders. They also realized that it was wrong to blame individuals living in squalid conditions beyond their control. Instead, stopping outbreaks requires cooperation among nations. With this in mind, postwar planners looked for ways to share medical information and new techniques in treatment. In 1919 health experts organized an international bureau to marshal global medical forces against epidemics. In 1946 that bureau led to the creation of the World Health Organization. The group's constitution set out its credo: "The enjoyment of the highest attainable standard of health is one of the fundamental rights of every human being without distinction of race, religion, political belief, economic or social condition."[31] Today the World Health Organization—despite many controversies—has led efforts to fight the COVID-19 pandemic, the deadliest global outbreak since the Spanish flu.

Political Fallout from the Pandemic

As the Spanish flu began to subside in the United States and Europe, its third wave slammed into Japan, Asia, and African nations. By then the disease had infected an estimated one-third of the world's population. From 50 million to 100 million people lost their lives to the flu worldwide, many more than died in World War I. The United States alone suffered about 675,000 deaths. In Africa, health care failures of the colonial system run by the European powers sparked resentment among the people. Seeds of rebellion had already been planted in India, Egypt, Kenya, and other British possessions. The Spanish flu may also have helped destabilize Europe in the 1930s. A 2020 study by the Federal Reserve Bank of New York suggests that the disease's ravages were an important factor in the rise of fascism and the Nazi Party in Germany. Its disruptions also doubtless played a part in the Russian Revolution, for which fighting continued into the early 1920s. As scientists and historians continue to study the Spanish flu and its fallout, their work may reveal pitfalls that await the modern world.

"The enjoyment of the highest attainable standard of health is one of the fundamental rights of every human being without distinction of race, religion, political belief, economic or social condition."[31]

—From the constitution of the World Health Organization

SOURCE NOTES

Introduction: The Deadliest Flu Outbreak in History

1. Elizabeth Hanink, "Nursing During the Spanish Flu Epidemic of 1918," Working Nurse, 2021. www.working nurse.com.
2. Quoted in Sara Francis Fujimara, "Purple Death: The Great Flu of 1918," *Perspectives in Health Magazine* 8, no. 3, 2003. www.paho.org.
3. Quoted in Teddy Amenabar, "'The 1918 Flu Is Still with Us': The Deadliest Pandemic Ever Is Still Causing Problems Today," *Washington Post*, September 3, 2020. www.washingtonpost.com.

Chapter One: A Pandemic Arises at the Great War's End

4. Quoted in World War I Document Archive, "Wilson's War Message to Congress," May 29, 2009. https://wwi.lib .byu.edu.
5. Quoted in Berkeley Lovelace Jr., "Medical Historian Compares the Coronavirus to the 1918 Flu Pandemic: Both Were Highly Political," CNBC, September 28, 2020. www.cnbc.com.
6. Quoted in Teddy Amenabar, "'The 1918 Flu Is Still with Us': The Deadliest Pandemic Ever Is Still Causing Problems Today," *Washington Post*, September 3, 2020. www.washingtonpost.com.
7. Quoted in Douglas Jordan, "Ask a CDC Scientist: Dr. Terrence Tumpey and the Reconstruction of the 1918 Pandemic Virus," Centers for Disease Control and Prevention, May 24, 2018. www.cdc.gov.
8. Quoted in Robert Roos, "Study: First Flu Wave in 1918 Was Vaccine for Some," Center for Infectious Disease Research and Policy, October 2, 2008. www.cidrap .umn.edu.

9. Quoted in Dave Roos, "Why the Second Wave of the 1918 Flu Pandemic Was So Deadly," *History*, December 22, 2020. www.history.com.

10. Quoted in Sarah Newey, "Could Sars-Cov-2 Be Evolving to Become More Transmissible—but Less Lethal?," *The Telegraph* (London), December 23, 2020. www.telegraph.co.uk.

Chapter Two: A Deadly Second Wave

11. Quoted in Nicholas Deshais, "The Doctor and the Pandemic: Spokane's 1918 Fight Against the Spanish Influenza," *Spokesman-Review* (Spokane, WA), January 20, 2019. www.spokesman.com.

12. Quoted in *American Experience*, "A Letter from Camp Devens," PBS. www.pbs.org.

13. Quoted in John Galvin, "Spanish Flu Pandemic: 1918," *Popular Mechanics*, July 31, 2007. www.popularmechanics.com.

14. Quoted in Patsy Widakuswara, "How US Presidents Have Handled Public Health Crises," VOA, March 30, 2020. www.voanews.com.

15. Quoted in Erik Lacitis, "As Coronavirus Spreads in 2020, Here's How Seattle Handled the 1918 Flu That Killed 1,513 People," *Seattle (WA) Times*, March 13, 2020. www.seattletimes.com.

16. Quoted in Mike Wallace, "How New York Survived the Great Pandemic of 1918," *New York Times*, March 20, 2020. www.nytimes.com.

17. Quoted in Piper Hudspeth Blackburn, "Obey the Laws, and Wear the Gauze: A Glance at Mask-Wearing in the US," Northwestern/Medill, April 21, 2020. https://nationalsecurityzone.medill.northwestern.edu.

Chapter Three: The Spanish Flu Becomes a Global Catastrophe

18. Quoted in Josh Jones, "*Dr. Wise on Influenza*: Rare Silent Film Shows How They Tried to Educate the Public About the Spanish Flu a Century Ago (1919)," Open Culture, July 20, 2020. www.openculture.com.

19. Quoted in BBC, "Coronavirus: How They Tried to Curb Spanish Flu Pandemic in 1918," May 10, 2020. www.bbc.com.

20. Quoted in James Thomas, "History Rhymes: Two Prime Ministers, Two Pandemics," Medium, April 13, 2020. https://mcdreeamie.medium.com.

21. Quoted in JF Ptak Science Books, "Beef Fat, Bones, and the Flu (1918)." https://longstreet.typepad.com.
22. Quoted in Jon King, "Armistice 100: 'Death and Misery' at Home as the War Guns Fall Silent," *Barking & Dagenham Post* (London), October 14, 2020. www.barkinganddagen hampost.co.uk.
23. Quoted in Maura Chhun, "1918 Flu Pandemic Killed 12 Million Indians, and British Overlords' Indifference Strengthened the Anti-colonial Movement," The Conversation, April 23, 2020. www.theconversation.com.
24. Laura Spinney, "Vital Statistics: How the Spanish Flu of 1918 Changed India," *The Caravan*, October 18, 2018. https://caravanmagazine.in.
25. Quoted in James Stout, "How American Samoa Kept a Pandemic at Bay," *Lapham's Quarterly*, April 2, 2020. www.laphamsquarterlly.org.

Chapter Four: The End and Aftereffects

26. Quoted in Eric Johnston, "A Century Later, Spanish Flu Pandemic Still Holds Valuable Lessons for Japanese and Global Health Experts," *Japan Times* (Tokyo), May 8, 2019. www.japantimes.co.jp.
27. Quoted in Fred Andayi, "How the Spanish Flu Affected Kenya—and Its Similarities to Coronavirus," The Conversation, April 22, 2020. www.theconversation.com.
28. Quoted in T.E. McMorrow, "1919: Influenza Enters Third Wave," *Dan's Papers*, May 19, 2020. www.danspapers.com.
29. Quoted in Ned Rozell, "How an Alaska Village Grave Led to a Spanish Flu Breakthrough," *Anchorage (AK) Daily News*, March 23, 2020. www.adn.com.
30. Douglas Jordan, "The Deadliest Flu: The Complete Story of the Discovery and Reconstruction of the 1918 Pandemic Virus," Centers for Disease Control and Prevention, December 17, 2019. www.cdc.gov.
31. Quoted in Laura Spinney, "How the 1918 Flu Pandemic Revolutionized Public Health," *Smithsonian*, September 27, 2017. www.smithsonianmag.com.

Books

Catharine Arnold, *Pandemic 1918: Eyewitness Accounts from the Greatest Medical Holocaust in Modern History.* New York: St. Martin's Griffin, 2018.

John M. Barry, *The Great Influenza: The Story of the Deadliest Pandemic in History.* New York: Penguin Books, 2018.

Jeremy Brown, *Influenza: The Hundred-Year Hunt to Cure the Deadliest Disease in History.* New York: Simon & Schuster, 2018.

Kenneth C. Davis, *More Deadly than War: The Hidden History of the Spanish Flu and the First World War.* New York: Holt, 2018.

Laura Spinney, *Pale Rider: The Spanish Flu of 1918 and How It Changed the World.* New York: Hachette, 2017.

Internet Sources

Teddy Amenabar, "'The 1918 Flu Is Still with Us': The Deadliest Pandemic Ever Is Still Causing Problems Today," *Washington Post*, September 3, 2020. www.washingtonpost.com.

Christine Crudo Blackburn et al., "How the 1918 Flu Pandemic Helped Advance Women's Rights," *Smithsonian*, March 2, 2018. www.smithsonianmag.com.

John Galvin, "Spanish Flu Pandemic: 1918," *Popular Mechanics*, July 31, 2007. www.popularmechanics.com.

Berkeley Lovelace Jr., "Medical Historian Compares the Coronavirus to the 1918 Flu Pandemic: Both Were Highly Political," CNBC, September 28, 2020. www.cnbc.com.

Ned Rozell, "How an Alaska Village Grave Led to a Spanish Flu Breakthrough," *Anchorage (AK) Daily News*, March 23, 2020. www.adn.com.

Websites

Centers for Disease Control and Prevention (CDC) (www .cdc.gov). The CDC works around the clock to protect America from health, safety, and security threats, both foreign and in the United States. Besides information about pandemics, including COVID-19, the CDC website contains a section on the Spanish flu, including a detailed look at how the virus was isolated and genetically reconstructed in a laboratory.

History (www.history.com). History provides an excellent source of information on world history. The website includes a variety of articles about the Spanish flu written by historians such as Christopher Klein's "How America Struggled to Bury the Dead During the 1918 Flu Pandemic." It also features many photographs and eyewitness accounts from the pandemic.

Influenza Encyclopedia (www.influenzaarchive.org). The Influenza Encyclopedia is the most comprehensive digital archive of historical documents about the Spanish flu. It was created by the University of Michigan Center for the History of Medicine and Michigan Publishing. Contemporary news articles cover every aspect of the Spanish flu pandemic, from government responses to medical treatments.

1914–1918 Online: International Encyclopedia of the First World War (https://encyclopedia.1914-1918-online.net). 1914–1918 Online covers every aspect of World War I, including how the war helped spread the deadly Spanish flu. This site has separate articles on Spanish flu outbreaks in different countries and regions in 1918 and afterward.

INDEX

PICTURE CREDITS